The 5-Minute Mind Reset

A BUSY PERSON'S GUIDE TO CALM & CLARITY

Frieda B.May

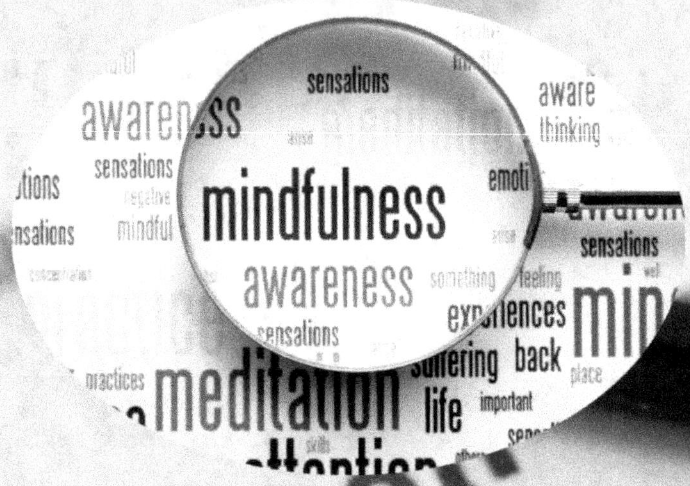
sensations
awareness
sensations
negative
mindful
mindfulness
awareness
emoti
sensations
aware
thinking
sensations
something
feeling
experiences
suffering back
meditation life important
attention
mindfulness
awareness
something
expe
suff

TABLE OF CONTENTS

Overwhelmed and limited on time? Discover the life-changing power of 5-minute morning mindfulness – unleash focus and resilience for a tranquil day. Modern existence rarely permits for hours of silent contemplation. This book is your shortcut to the transformative benefits of mindfulness, offering brief, practical meditations designed for even the busiest mornings. Learn to break free from mental overwhelm, tap into a wellspring of focus, and develop the inner strength to manage life's challenges with greater ease.

This book understands the unique challenges of modern existence. Forget protracted meditation retreats or vague promises of immediate enlightenment. Instead, you'll discover the transformative power of brief, targeted practices integrated seamlessly into your busy routine.

Inside, you'll find:

- The Why and How of Mindfulness: A clear summary of what mindfulness is, its neuroscience-backed benefits, and how to dispel common misconceptions keeping you trapped.

- Your Guided Meditations: Step-by-step weekly meditations concentrating on breath awareness, body scans, embracing

thoughts and emotions, and cultivating compassion – the
pillars of a potent mindfulness practice.

- Beyond the Cushion: Practical suggestions on integrating
  mindfulness into your everyday life, from mindful moments
  at work to walking meditations for increased focus and well-
  being.

- Troubleshooting and Growth: Anticipating common
  challenges, this book offers support and encouragement to
  cultivate a sustainable practice.

"5-Minute Guided Morning Mindfulness Meditation" is more than a
book; it's an invitation to rediscover peace, clarity, and pleasure –
even with a jam-packed schedule. Whether you're a stressed-out
parent, an overburdened professional, or simply seeking more calm,
these five-minute sessions hold the potential to transform your life
from   the   inside   out.

YOUR MINDFULNESS MOMENT STARTS NOW

Imagine your life as a busy train station. Thoughts run in and out like fast trains. Emotions steam and chug, adding to the commotion. Stress hangs heavy in the air, a constant rush hour. You're stuck on the platform, caught in the blur, wishing for a moment of stillness.

This is the experience of the modern mind – overbooked, overwhelmed, and wanting a stop button. We all know we should be more aware, and less impulsive. But in a world demanding constant attention, where does someone with a jam-packed schedule even begin?

What if I told you that recovering a sense of calm doesn't take hours on a meditation cushion or a retreat to a mountain monastery? What if finding a sliver of peace amidst the chaos could be as easy as giving five minutes each morning to yourself?

That's the power of "5-Minute Guided Morning Mindfulness Meditations". This little book is your ticket to a less stressed, more focused, and surprisingly happy existence. Whether you're a stressed-out professional, a harried parent, or anyone juggling too many tasks, you have the time for this.

Mindfulness: Not Just Trendy, but Transformative

You've probably heard the awareness talk. It's not just a fad; it's a well-researched practice with real effects. Scientific studies show that regular mindfulness practice can:

- Melt away stress: It re-wires your brain's stress response, helping you to handle pressure with more ease.

- Sharpen your focus: Think of it as a mental workout, improving your ability to focus and tune out distractions.

- Boost your mood: Mindfulness promotes self-compassion, which combats anxiety and enhances general well-being.

- Improve decision-making: Helps you step back from automatic responses and make decisions from a place of understanding.

The best part? These perks aren't limited to monks or yoga teachers. With constant practice, even in short bursts, mindfulness can change your relationship with your mind.

Why Mornings Matter

While you can fit in a mindfulness micro-session anytime, mornings are a game-changer. Think of it as preventative care for your day. Before emails, meetings, and the expected curveballs life throws your way, you carve out a few minutes to center yourself.

This sets the tone for greater composure and resolve as you manage the hours ahead.

No Prior Experience Necessary

If words like "empty your mind" or "achieve enlightenment" make you want to run for the hills, relax. This isn't about becoming a meditation guru. We're looking for growth, not perfection.

Forget trying to force your mind into zen-like blankness. Mindfulness is simply about learning to watch your present experience – the jumbled thoughts, the restless urges, the background hum of the body – with gentle curiosity and without judgment. It's about being present, right here, right now.

And what could be easier than just five minutes of being present?

The 5-Minute Advantage

In our drive for instant satisfaction, five minutes seems insignificant. But remember, constancy is key. A tiny daily practice builds into amazing power over time. It's the difference between an occasional splash of water and steady rain changing a parched area.

These guided meditations are meant for maximum effect with minimal time investment. No difficult methods to master, no esoteric jargon to learn. You'll be led step-by-step with clear instructions and gentle reminders to keep your attention.

An Invitation to Transformation

Consider this book your guide to the world of mindfulness, specially tailored for those with limited time and no previous experience. Within these pages, you'll discover:

The basics of awareness and its science-backed benefits

- How to find those valuable five minutes and create a consistent morning routine

- Simple but powerful guided meditations designed to fit easily into your busy schedule

- Troubleshooting tips for problems you may face

- Ways to extend mindfulness beyond the five-minute exercise and reap its benefits throughout your day

Are you ready to trade five minutes of frantic reading or mindless snoozing for a quieter, more focused version of yourself? Let's start this journey together. Your moment of inner stillness awaits.

OPEN
MIND
mental
focusing
bodily
sensation
mindfulness
achieved

WHAT IS MINDFULNESS?

Simple definition: giving attention to the present moment without judgment

This seemingly simple definition holds the key to a profound shift in how we connect with our own experience. Let's unpack it:

- Paying attention: At its core, mindfulness is about actively directing our awareness. It's an active process, a kind of mental lighting that we focus on a chosen target.

- To the present: The only time we can truly occupy is now. Yet, so often our minds are lost in thinking about the past or worried about projecting into the future. Mindfulness draws us back to the intensity of this moment, with all its feelings, thoughts, and emotions.

- Without judgment: Our default mode is often to name and rate everything we experience. "This feeling is good, that one is bad. This thought is important, that one's stupid." Mindfulness asks us to stop those automatic conclusions and simply watch with curiosity. It's not about accepting or rejecting, just noticing.

How Mindfulness Differs from Regular Thinking

The mind is a thought-generating machine. It never truly shuts off. However, our everyday way of thought tends to be:

- Distracted: We bounce from one thought to the next, following associations and memory trails, pulled by outward events. Think of a fly moving from object to object in a messy room.

- Narrative-driven: Our thoughts often build stories about ourselves, others, and the world. We cling to these tales, reading reality through the lens of our past experiences and biases.

- Problem-focused: The mind's normal habit is to focus on what's wrong, scanning for possible threats or dwelling on regrets. This puts us on edge and robs us of fun.

- Auto-pilot: A large amount of our thoughts are habitual, repeated, and unconscious. We rarely stop to question the truth or helpfulness of these thought loops.

Mindfulness calls us to step out of this habitual, reactive mode and into a more conscious and observational connection with our inner world. Here's a breakdown of the key differences:

Regular Thinking vs. Mindfulness

Characteristic	Regular Thinking	Mindfulness
Focus	Chaotic, unfocused, easily distracted	Intentional, directed to a chosen object of awareness
Relationship to Present	Often focusing on the past or thinking about the future	Grounded in the here and now, the immediate experience
Attitude	Judgmental, labeling things as good/bad, pleasant/unpleasant	Non-judgmental, observing with curiosity and acceptance
Mode of Processing	Narrative-driven, focused on stories	Experiential, attuned to raw

	and interpretations	sensations, thoughts, emotions
Degree of Awareness	Automatic, "living in our heads"	Conscious, actively noticing our inner and outer world

Imagine your thoughts and feelings as clouds moving across the sky. Regular thinking means getting caught up in the clouds – connecting with them, worrying about their shapes, getting swept away by them. Mindfulness offers the view of the sky – vast, clear, and constant. The clouds (thoughts and feelings) still come and go, but you realize that you are not the clouds themselves. You are the place that holds them.

Benefits of this Shift

Cultivating this mindful awareness isn't just about feeling less stressed, though that's surely a nice benefit. Mindfulness offers a number of changing possibilities:

- Freedom from thought chatter: You begin to see that you don't have to believe or respond to every thought that pops into your head. This makes room for wiser decisions instead of knee-jerk reactivity.

- Emotional regulation: By non-judgmentally watching feelings, we understand their transient nature. They rise and fall without completely swallowing us.

- Increased self-awareness: Mindfulness shows tiny inner processes, habits, and biases we might not otherwise notice. This allows us to make good changes.

- Enhanced compassion: The practice of non-judgment stretches towards ourselves and others. We become less harsh in our self-criticism and more patient with those around us.

Importantly, the difference between regular thought and mindfulness isn't about turning off our mind. It's about cultivating a new connection to our mental activity, acknowledging its power but not being dominated by it

Why Do We Need It?

In today's fast-paced, hyper-connected world, our minds rarely have a chance to slow down. Technology bombards us with stimuli, social standards pull us in multiple ways, and the pressure to achieve leads to relentless inner trying. The effects of this nonstop mental churn are important.

The Nonstop Mind and Its Pitfalls

In the modern world, our thoughts rarely get a break. We're flooded with information, alerts, and an endless stream of to-dos. Even when trying to relax, we scroll, binge-watch, or endlessly ponder. This constant brain activity takes a toll.

- Stress: The Overload Effect Our brains evolved to handle acute worry – the burst of adrenaline needed to avoid an attacker. However, chronic, low-level stress from constant expectations becomes toxic. We're constantly in a state of fight-or-flight, with no down-regulation in sight. This affects our physical and mental health deeply.

- Anxiety: Caught in the Worry Loops Our brains have a negativity bias, scanning for risks even when none are present. When that survival tool goes into overdrive, it leads to widespread anxiety – racing thoughts, anticipatory fear, and trouble finding calm.

- Autopilot Mode: Mindlessly Going Through the Motions Much of our behavior and decision-making runs on autopilot – ingrained habits and shortcuts to save mental energy. While helpful sometimes, we become enslaved to habit, unable to step out of self-sabotaging patterns or see new views.

THE NEUROSCIENCE BEHIND MINDFULNESS

While these challenges may feel purely psychological, they have clear physical footprints in our brains. Luckily, neuroscience shows that mindfulness training isn't just about feeling a bit better; it literally rewires the processes involved in stress, attention, and mood. Here's how:

- Taming the Amygdala: This almond-shaped brain area is our fire warning system, kicking off the stress reaction. Mindfulness practice improves the link between the amygdala and the prefrontal cortex (the rational, planning part of our brain). This allows us to down-regulate our reactions and see events more clearly before losing our cool.

- Growing the Attention Muscle: Mindfulness builds up parts of the brain responsible for attentional focus. Like flexing a muscle, our ability to consciously direct and hold our concentration improves with practice. We become less easily sidetracked by outward pulls or our mental chatter.

- Calming the Monkey Mind: Regions involved in the 'default mode network', responsible for self-referential thought and mind wandering, quiet down through meditation. That constant self-centered narrative? You start to experience gaps in it, times of peaceful present.

- Increased Neuroplasticity: Mindfulness supports neuroplasticity, the brain's ability to form new links and change. This gives us more flexibility in our reactions and allows us to change limiting thought habits and behaviors.

The Cumulative Effects

These brain changes translate into real benefits in our daily lives:

- Stress Resilience: You don't become immune to trials, but your nervous system finds a calmer baseline. It's like the difference between a small pebble causing waves in a still pond vs. throwing a boulder into a stormy ocean.

- Emotional Equanimity: Mindfulness helps you watch feelings emerge and fall without getting controlled by them. You're less likely to get swept away by impulsive anger, brief sadness, or crushing fear.

- Breaking Out of Autopilot: Increased awareness lets you see where habits are helping you and where they're not. You regain conscious choice instead of mindlessly repeating old habits.

- Self-Compassion & Wisdom: With less sharp inner judgment, space opens up for understanding and kindness towards yourself and others. This, in turn, leads to wiser choices aligned with your ideals.

Important Notes:

- Mindfulness isn't a magic bullet. It takes practice and sometimes uncomfortable self-observation. However, the benefits are well worth the work.

- This isn't against current technology. There's nothing fundamentally wrong with our fast-paced world. Mindfulness offers tools to handle it with better sanity and well-being.

- Science offers support, not approval. You don't need to understand neuroscience to gain awareness. However, understanding that there's a scientific base can boost the drive for those initially skeptical.

Mindfulness enables us to reclaim our thoughts and experience greater resilience, clarity, and ease in a world driven to pull us in a thousand directions.

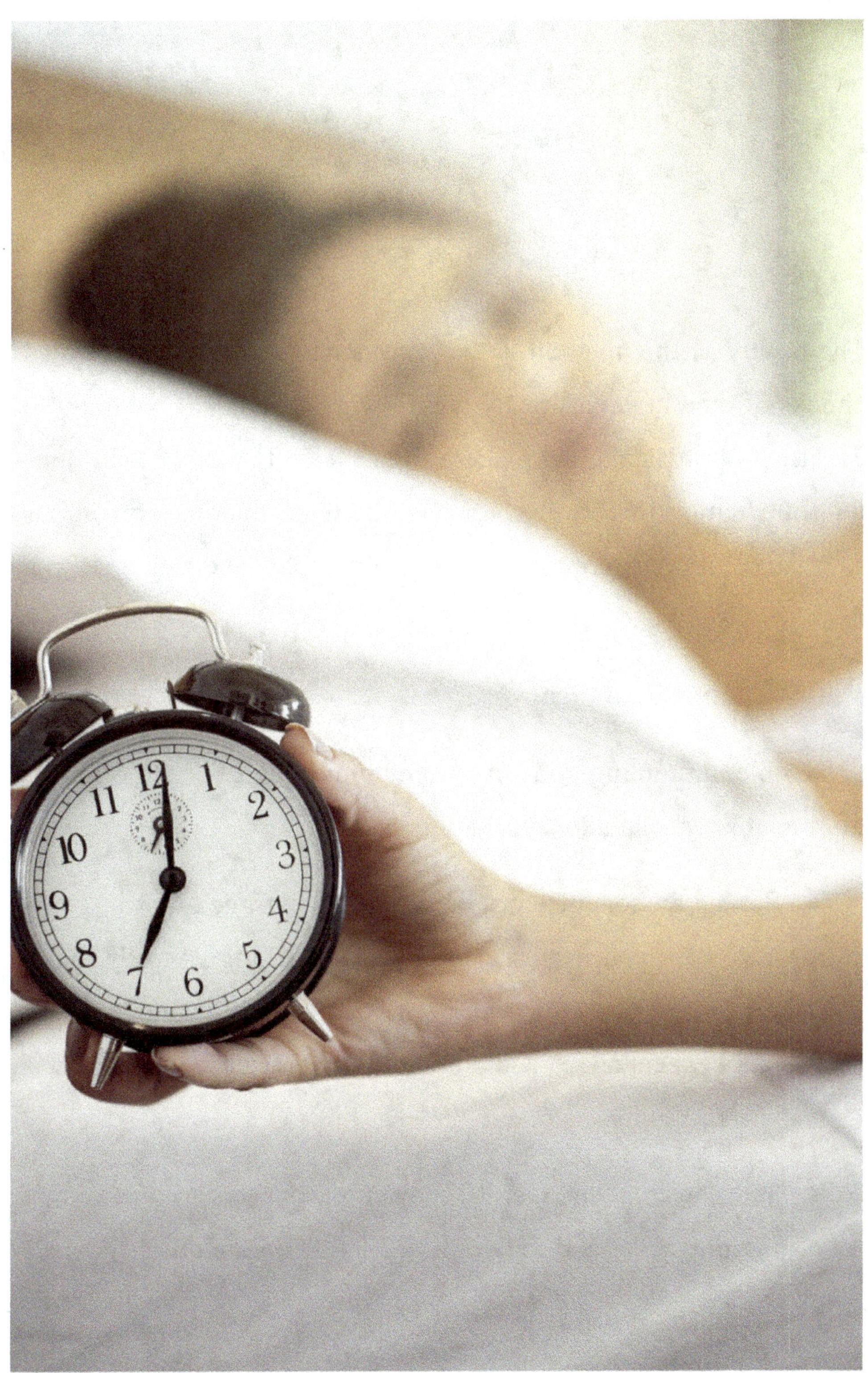

FINDING YOUR 5 MINUTES

The beauty of this method is that you don't need to clear out huge chunks of time in your already overflowing schedule. Five minutes, consistently, are going to make a bigger effect than the odd hour-long meditation that rarely happens due to competing obligations. Let's study how to improve those five minutes and where to find them.

Why Mornings Are Ideal

If possible, grounding your five-minute mindfulness exercise in the morning has special advantages:

- Setting the tone: Before the relentless barrage of to-dos, messages, and requests starts, you are gifting yourself a few minutes of conscious calm. This primes you to handle the day's expected ups and downs with more self-awareness and less reactivity.

- Willpower advantage: Willpower tends to be stronger in the morning. By handling your meditation before other choices and tasks begin draining your supplies, you're more likely to follow through.

- Preempting the mental snowball: We all know how our thoughts can quickly spin up throughout the day, making it more difficult to find stillness in the evening. A morning practice offers a proactive reset button.

Now, this doesn't mean you're doomed if mornings are absolutely crazy for you. The driving principle is finding a pocket of time that you can truly protect and make your awareness center. It could be:

- Right after waking up: Before diving into emails or reading social media, commit those first five minutes to a guided mindfulness exercise.

- Your commute: If you drive or take public transportation, try turning off the radio and practicing easy breath awareness instead. (For safety, if driving, focus on body feelings while keeping your eyes open or practice at stoplights).

- Coffee/tea break: Instead of idly sipping, turn those five minutes into a focused tea meditation: noticing the warmth, aroma, and flavors.

- Lunch break: Step away from your work (and screens!). Mindfully walk outside for a few minutes, feeling the sun on your face, and watching the trees.

- Right before bed: This can be helpful for 'switching off' a busy mind and promoting better sleep. Choose a relaxation-focused meditation.

Micro-Meditations Throughout the Day

Beyond your main five-minute practice, micro-meditations spread widely throughout the day can boost the benefits you experience. Think of these as little brain power-ups:

- Waiting in line: Instead of angrily moving, bring your attention to your feet on the ground, and take a few deep, aware breaths.

- Transitioning between tasks: Instead of barreling from one thing to the next, stop for 30 seconds and feel your body sitting in the chair, your hands on the computer. This produces small "reset" times.

- Before answering the phone or a difficult email: Take one mindful breath, leaving a short gap between stimulus and response, which can avoid rash or overemotional responses.

Consistency Over Duration

It's more important to develop the habit of a short, daily exercise than to try meditating for an extended time sporadically. Here's an analogy: watering a plant with a small amount of water every day does wonders; occasionally soaking it and then neglecting it for weeks results in a droopy, unhappy plant.

How to focus five minutes when faced with real-life hurdles:

- The 'No-Matter-What' mindset: There will be some days when even five minutes might feel like a stretch. In that case, shoot for even one minute of aware breathing, a mindful walk around the block, or a 30-second pause while washing your hands. Every little bit counts, and it keeps the energy you've been building.

- Make it enjoyable: Don't view it as a job. Choose guided meditations with a voice and style you find soothing. Practice in a place that brings a sense of peace, even if it's just a comfortable chair on your porch.

- Don't judge your practice: Some days your attention will be laser-sharp, others your mind will be filled with talk. That's normal! Gently re-focus when you become distracted. The act of noticing the distraction and getting back to your chosen center is where the mindfulness practice truly lies.

- Be patient: You are building a new skill; the results will unfold gradually. Instead of chasing specific states of happiness, approach each practice with fun and curiosity. What do you notice in your body and your mind? How does this present moment feel?

This method turns those spare times throughout the day into chances to strengthen your relationship with conscious awareness. It starts with making a conscious choice to pause, take a breath, and watch – again and again, and again.

CREATING A SUPPORTIVE SPACE

While mindfulness is ultimately about awareness of the present moment wherever you are, making a dedicated place for your practice can be incredibly helpful, especially in the beginning. Think of it as making a nest for your mind—a calm haven away from the pressures of the outside world.

The Importance of a Quiet Corner

The biggest hurdle to developing focused awareness is usually distraction. In our noisy, device-driven lives, areas of true quiet are rare. Aim to find a corner of your home where you can sit quietly for at least five minutes of practice.

Here's what makes a good mindfulness spot:

- Relative silence: While total soundproofing is a luxury, try to choose a place free from sudden noises, loud electronics, or chatty roommates. If outdoor noise is unavoidable, earplugs or gentle background music can mask some of it.

- Limited visible clutter: A busy and messy environment makes it harder for your mind to settle. Find a spot with clear surfaces and simple settings. It doesn't need to be clean, but a sense of tidiness is helpful.

- Privacy: This might mean training before the rest of the household wakes up, using a bathroom stall when moving, or simply asking your family for five minutes of uninterrupted time. You'll focus better knowing you won't be interrupted.

Minimizing Distractions

Even in a quiet area, distractions can creep in. Taking a few easy steps will create a haven conducive to focus:

- Airplane mode: Silence your phone, smartwatch, and any other tool with alerts. The world won't end in those five minutes – consider it a short digital break.

- Close the door: This is both a real and psychological barrier. It signals to your mind – and others – that it's time to turn inward.

- Dim the lights (optional): If possible, lowering the light level can gently improve a feeling of calmness and introspection.

- Harness nature: Sitting near a window with a view of trees or sky can support rest. Indoor plants add a calm natural touch.

Note: Your mindfulness place doesn't have to be forever. If life gets busy, change! Practice on a blanket in a quiet park during your lunch break, or set a timer for five minutes in your stopped car before going to work. The freedom is part of making this practice truly effective.

Comfortable but Alert Posture

Posture plays a vital part in mindfulness practice, touching both our physical comfort and mental attention. The standard meditation position may come to mind: sitting cross-legged on a cushion with a perfectly straight spine. However, this isn't necessary, especially for short training! Remember, the goal is finding a position that keeps you relaxed but standing enough to avoid drowsiness. Let's explore the options:

- Seated on a chair: Choose a sturdy chair that lets your feet rest flat on the floor. Your spine should be naturally upright, without trying to keep a perfect posture. A small cushion put on your lower back can provide extra support.

- Cross-legged on the floor: If you're comfortable sitting this way, a cushion or folded blanket under your hips will help in proper spine alignment. It's fine if your knees aren't touching the floor.

- Kneeling: Consider a meditation bench or cushion as support. This lowers hip flexibility demands and helps keep alertness.

- Lying down (with caution): Mindfulness exercise while lying down is possible, but the main risk is falling asleep! If you know you're prone to this, stick to a seated position to develop attentional alertness.

Here are key rules for good posture during meditation:

- Stable base: Whether sitting or standing, have a sense of being rooted to the ground, supported by the surface below.

- Effortless straightness: Find a balance between a tight, forced stance and falling. Imagine your spine extending upwards naturally like a stack of building blocks.

- Relaxed shoulders: Let your shoulders drop away from your ears, releasing needless stress.

- Resting hands: You can fold your hands gently in your lap, or let them rest on your knees or legs. Choose what feels most comfortable.

Beyond the Basics: Personalizing Your Space

While not exactly required, a couple of small additions can enhance the ambiance of your exercise area. These are highly personal touches, so go with what works for you:

- Soothing objects: A candle, a plant, or a beautiful picture can help you make a calming visual focus. Avoid anything overly busy or exciting.

- Scents: A light touch of incense or essential oils can add to a sense of calm if you find them pleasing. Choose mild, natural smells.

- Comfort items: A cozy blanket for those chilly mornings can encourage the body to relax, allowing for greater mental resting.

Remember, perfection isn't the goal. Find what works for you, with the tools you have.

The most important thing is to avoid causing pain or soreness. If a posture hurts, slowly change until you find greater ease. It's far better to have a more comfortable stance that helps awareness than a 'perfect' position that leaves you aching and distracted.

While the essence of mindfulness needs nothing more than your focused attention, certain tools can be incredibly helpful, especially as you're starting your practice. Think of them as training wheels – supportive at first, but not strictly required as your awareness muscles get stronger. Here's a look at some useful options:

Meditation Cushions/Chairs

The Goal: Finding a comfy but aware position. This is key to escaping the twin pitfalls of falling asleep and fidgeting from physical pain.

Traditional Cushions: These come in different forms. Popular choices include:

- Zafu: A round, firm cushion giving good height and support.

- Zabuton: A larger, padded mat put under the zafu for extra support on knees and feet.

- Crescent/Gomden: These curved cushions make a gentle slope, helpful if you have tight hips or lower back problems.

- Chairs: If sitting cross-legged causes too much pain, don't force it. A sturdy chair allows for an upright spine, feet flat on the floor, and hands gently sitting on your lap or legs.

Additional Supports: If needed, rolled-up blankets or small cushions can offer back support or change seat height. The right support lets your body relax so that your mind can focus on the meditation.

What to Look For

- Firmness: Enough support to keep your back straight without sinking in too much.

- Height: Choose a height that supports proper posture: hips are slightly above knees for cushions, with the spine easily erect.

- Comfort: It's important to find something that doesn't cause distracting pain or discomfort. Experiment with different styles to find what feels best for your body.

Apps and Guided Meditations

Perfect for Beginners: Guided exercises are an excellent way to learn the ropes. Hearing directions takes the guesswork out of what to do and keeps you on track.

Variety is Key: Numerous apps offer guided exercises of various lengths, focusing on different methods (breath awareness, body scan, loving-kindness, etc.). Experiment to find sounds and styles that connect with you. Popular choices include:

- Headspace: User-friendly, playful beginning classes, and a huge library of themed exercises.

- Calm: Beautiful nature images, focus on relaxation and sleep exercises.

- Insight Timer: Vast collection of guided meditations from different teachers and traditions.

- Ten Percent Happier: Combines guided meditations with understandable descriptions of mindfulness ideas.

Choosing an App:

- Voice: Does the voice of the storyteller feel nice or irritating? This makes a big difference.

- Style: Some apps have long introductory progressions; others favor a more 'drop-in' method. Explore styles to see what clicks for you.

- Free vs. Paid: Many apps have a simple free offering to get a feel before paying.

Going Beyond the Guided: While it's fine to rely on guided exercises for a long time, consider adding times of unguided practice where you simply watch your breath or whatever your chosen center is. This builds self-reliance in your awareness exercise.

Soothing Background Sounds

- Masking Distractions: For settings with uncertain noise, soothing sounds can create a tranquil bubble for your exercise. Gentle waves, rain sounds, or soft instrumental music are popular picks.

- Supporting Deep Relaxation: Specific sound frequencies are thought to help reduce anxiousness and create calmer brainwave states. Binaural beats or sound therapy tracks are worth trying if relaxation is your main goal.

- Important Caveat: Background noise should never fight for your attention. The goal is to subtly minimize distractions, not replace one topic with another. Find sounds that you can easily fade into the background.

Additional Notes on Tools

- No Need to Buy Everything: Start with what you have! A regular chair, free meditation apps, and a quiet area are perfectly suited. As your business deepens, you can invest in specialized tools if they offer real benefits.

- Don't Get Attached: Ultimately, mindfulness is about being present with what is, without having anything external. The props are good, but remember, the true training happens within.

- Rituals Matter: The simple act of arranging your cushion, taking a mindful seat, and playing your chosen music can signal to your mind and body that it's time to stop and be present. This consistency improves the efficiency of your exercise.

Important Considerations

Finding the right tools for your work is unique and may take some testing. Here's a plan to help you:

- Comfort: Does your chosen setup allow you to keep an alert position without excessive pain or restlessness?

- Accessibility: Do your tools match your lifestyle and resources? A fancy meditation cushion is useless if it gets tucked away in the closet because you never have time to set it up.

- Sustainability: Is this something you can realistically see yourself using consistently? Choose choices that compliment your life, not complicate it.

The tools themselves are meant to gently fade into the background. With practice, the mere desire to meditate will be enough to trigger the deep focus and presence that are at the heart of mindfulness.

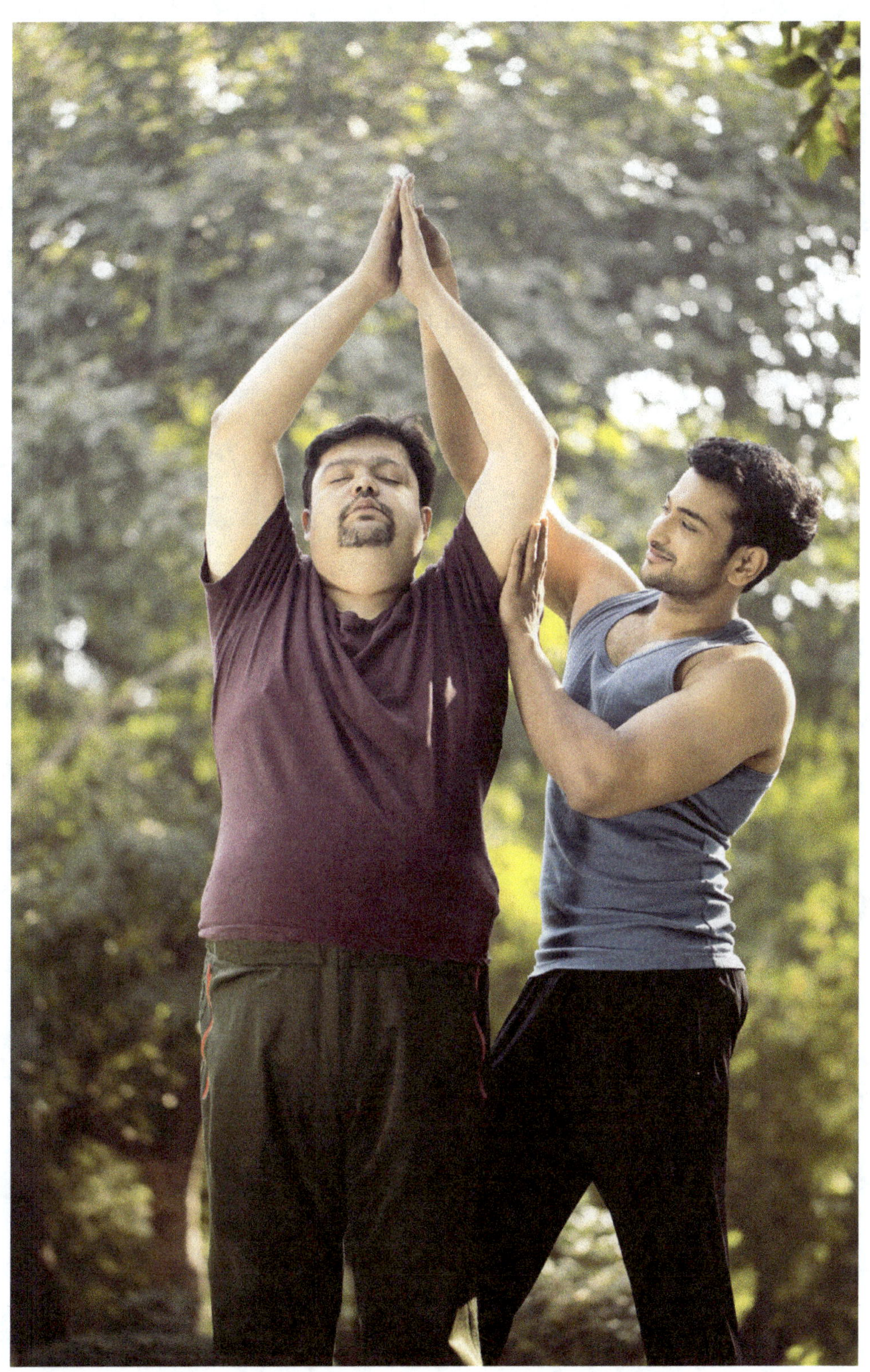

Week 1: The Breath as Anchor

Welcome to the practical heart of your mindfulness journey! This week is all about creating a simple yet strong foundation: using your breath as your awareness anchor.

Why the Breath?

The breath is both interesting and essential. Here's why it's the best object of focus for beginners:

- Always Available: Unlike external signs, your breath is a steady companion. No matter where you are or what you're doing, it's happening in the background.

- Connects Body and Mind: The breath has a physical component (the feelings of air going in and out) and a mental component (the thoughts and emotions we often attach to breathing). It acts as a bridge to link body and mind in the moment.

- Naturally Calming: When we pay attention to our breath, we tend to subconsciously deepen and control it. This triggers the parasympathetic nervous system, responsible for the "rest and digest" reaction and counteracting stress.

- Simple but Not Easy: Focusing on the breath seems easy enough, but you'll quickly learn how easily the mind gets sidetracked. This offers the perfect training ground to build mindfulness: patience, acceptance, and constantly re-directing attention.

The practices this week are incredibly simple in idea, yet mastering them takes time and care. Remember, the goal isn't to achieve perfect attention but to constantly practice noticing when your mind wanders and gently bringing it back. This act of non-judgmental returning is at the core of awareness.

Week 1: Basic Breath Awareness

- Find a comfy place. You can sit in a chair, on a cushion, or even lie down if that's most relaxing. The key is to keep a sense of awareness without feeling strained.

- Gently close your eyes, or leave them half-open with a soft look. Do whatever feels most comfortable.

- Feel your body. Bring your attention to the feelings of your body in touch with the chair or surface beneath you. Notice the weight of your body.

- Turn towards the breath. Without trying to change it, simply become aware of the natural flow of your inhales and exhales. It may be helpful to pick a single spot where you feel the breath most clearly –perhaps the nose, the rise and fall of your chest, or your belly.

- Just observe. Notice the inhale as it starts, the fullness of the breath, and the slow release of the exhale. There's no right or wrong way to do this – simply watch with interest.

- The wandering mind. Inevitably, your mind will wander. Thoughts will pop up, memories appear, or you might be sidetracked by sounds. When you notice, don't get upset! Gently recognize the thought or distraction without following it. Just name it internally with a word like "thinking" or "sound." Then, kindly guide your attention back to the breath.

- Again and again. This pattern of noticing distraction and returning to the breath is the heart of the exercise. Be patient with yourself. Start with just a few minutes, and gradually raise the length as you feel comfortable.

Day 2-3: Counting Breaths

This exercise adds a slight mental component to fix your attention even more strongly. Here's how:

- Follow the basic breath awareness directions from Day 1 to settle in.

- Start quietly counting your exhales: "One" on the first exhale, "Two" on the second, and so on.

- When you hit the count of ten, start back at one.

- If you lose track (and you will!), just start again at one. Don't judge yourself, gently restart. This act of beginning is the practice!

Day 4-7: Noticing Sensations

Broaden your awareness beyond simply following the breath's beat. See if you can notice smaller details:

- Temperature: Is the air cool entering your nose, warmer as you exhale?

- Expansion and contraction: Can you track the gentle movement of your chest or belly as you breathe?

- Subtle vibrations: Is there a weak tingling or buzzing feeling related to the breath anywhere in your body?

- The pause: As your exhale stops, there's a tiny pause before the next inhale starts. Can you feel this?

- Keep returning to these feelings whenever your mind slips. Let the breath be your leading light.

Tips for the First Week

- Consistency is key! Short daily exercise is far more helpful than longer, infrequent lessons.

- Don't seek perfection. There will be "good" days where you feel focused, and "bad" days where your mind runs wild. All are part of the process!

- Attitude is everything. Approach this with soft interest, not stiff self-criticism.

- Start with short sessions: As a beginner, 3-5 minutes of any of these routines is a great starting place. Gradually increase time as you get relaxed.

- Experiment and find what resonates: It's totally fine to find one exercise more settling than others.

- Be kind to yourself: This is called a 'practice' for a reason. Every time you bring your attention back to the breath after distraction, you're training your awareness muscle.

As you finish this week, you may already start to notice a slight shift in how you connect to your thoughts and the world around you. Keep building on this base!

WEEK 2: EMBRACING THE BODY

This week, we turn our mindful attention toward the amazing vessel that moves us through life – our physical body. Too often, we dwell solely in our heads, disconnected from the rich flow of bodily feelings. The body scan method is a powerful way to reconnect and cultivate a more grounded presence.

The Body Scan Technique

The body scan involves carefully focusing your attention on different areas of your body, from the tips of your toes to the crown of your head. The goal isn't to change anything but to simply tune in and notice whatever sensations are present – or even a lack of sensation. Here's a basic flow:

1. Settle In: Find a comfy position, either sitting or lying down. You can close your eyes or keep them softly open, fixed on an uncluttered spot.

2. Anchoring the Breath: Spend a few minutes feeling the natural flow of your breath. The physical feelings of inhaling and exhaling act as your anchor point.

3. Sequential Scan: Start by bringing your awareness to your toes, noticing any feelings of touch, pressure, temperature, or movement. Slowly move upward, moving to your feet, ankles, calves, knees, thighs, and so on. Spend a minute or two in each place, simply observing. Some parts might have distinct sensations, while others feel neutral. Notice it all without judgment.

4. Releasing and Softening: If you notice tension anywhere (the jaw, forehead, and shoulders are common culprits), actively release and soften those muscles. It can help to picture breathing into that area with each in-breath.

5. Whole Body Awareness: After reaching the top of your head, expand your awareness to take in your full body as a unified whole.

6. Patience and acceptance: It's normal for the mind to wander, especially at first. That's okay! The moment you realize you've become distracted, simply recognize it and guide your attention back to the body, without frustration. This process of noticing and gently returning is at the heart of mindfulness.

Releasing Tension

We store a surprising amount of stress in our bodies. The body scan becomes a tool for spotting and unclenching. Don't force relaxation; it's more about a gentle desire to let go. Remember, even fleeting times of released tension provide the body with much-needed rest.

Some Common Sensations You Might Notice:

- Tingling or warmth

- Tightness or pressure

- Throbbing or pulsing

- Vibrating or buzzing

- Itching

- Numbness or a feeling of absence

Observe them all with interest, but try not to label them as "good" or "bad." Simply meet each feeling with a "knowing" quality of awareness.

Grounding Yourself in the Present

The body is an ever-present link to the here and now. When the mind gets lost in worries or distractions, the simple act of noticing sensations in your feet, for example, roots you in the immediacy of this moment. This grounding offers steadiness and reduces a sense of mental or emotional overwhelm.

Benefits of the Body Scan

- Regular practice of the body scan helps:

- Reduce stress and anxiety: By tuning into physical sensations, we bring ourselves back to the present, interrupting cycles of rumination and fear.

- Improve sleep: Focusing on the body can quiet a racing mind, promoting relaxation and setting conditions for a good night's rest.

- Manage chronic pain: Mindfulness methods have been shown to lessen the perceived intensity of pain and improve coping mechanisms.

- Increase body awareness: We become more sensitive to cues the body sends, leading to better choices about self-care.

- Foster self-compassion: Non-judgmental observation of the body helps us accept ourselves as we are, flaws and all.

Sample Guidance for a Body Scan Meditation (for you to change or record)

Begin by finding an easy and supported position... Gently close your eyes, or find a soft resting point for your gaze...Take a few full, deep breaths, noticing your belly rising and falling...

Bring your attention to your toes... Notice any feelings there, tingling, pressure, or perhaps a sense of nothing at all... Let the toes simply be as they are...

Move your focus to the soles of your feet... Are they warm? Cool?... Is there a feeling of contact with the floor or your shoes?... Continue softening any tightness you notice...

(Proceed to guide the awareness upward, giving 1-2 minutes to each area: ankles, legs, knees, thighs, hips, lower back, belly, upper back, chest, shoulders, hands, arms, neck, jaw, face, top of the head) Finally, breathe into your body as a whole... Sensing the length, the weight, the space your body fills... Allow yourself to feel centered and supported...

Before opening your eyes, take a moment to recognize gratitude for this body, this extraordinary vessel that supports your life...

Tips for Effective Body Scans

- Regularity is key: Short, frequent body scans are more helpful than long, occasional ones. Even 5-10 minutes a day can make a noticeable change.

- Vary the pace: Some days, you might take a quick scan for a general check-in. On other days, spend more time with each body part, really exploring the nuanced sensations.

- Don't rush judgment: If you feel discomfort or pain, it's tempting to label it "bad" and tense up. Practice just noticing: "There's sharpness here," "A throbbing sensation."

- Compassion is key: Be kind to your body. This is not a performance, but a study of what is currently true.

The body scan is a powerful tool for cultivating a deeper relationship with your physical being, releasing tension, and finding calm within the ever-changing landscape of sensations.

By now, you've built a foundation with breath awareness and body scanning methods. You're getting comfortable with bringing gentle attention to the physical feelings of the present moment. This week, we expand our attention to the sometimes tumultuous landscape of thoughts and feelings.

Observing Thoughts Like Passing Clouds

Our minds are constantly producing thoughts – some important, some utterly absurd, some naggingly repetitive. This mental commentary can easily spiral into worry, rumination, or self-criticism. Week 3's practice teaches you to view thoughts with more detachment and less reactivity.

Here's the core mindfulness skill: understanding that you are not your thoughts. Thoughts are events happening in your mind, much like sounds occur in your surroundings. Just as you can be aware of traffic rumbling down the street without needing to follow every car, you can notice thoughts without getting swept away by them.

Let's review the metaphor of clouds and sky. Your thoughts are the ever-changing clouds. There will be windy days filled with dark, swirling clouds and days with just a few fluffy wisps. The goal isn't to control the weather in your thoughts but to remember you are the spacious sky that simply observes its changing conditions.

Guided Practice: Watching the Thought Stream

1. Settle into a comfortable position: Find your usual meditation spot and make an environment of quiet and minimal distraction.

2. Anchor in the breath: Begin with a few minutes of easy breath awareness. Notice the rising and falling of your belly, the rush of air at your nostrils. This roots you in the present moment.

3. Open the gates of awareness: Gradually widen your focus to include the flow of thoughts going through your mind. There's no need to examine or fixate on them. Just notice they are there.

4. Labeling with detachment: If it helps, quietly label your thoughts. "Thinking," "planning," "judging," "remembering."

This act of naming creates a bit of distance, telling you that thoughts are mental events, not defining truths about you.

5. Witnessing without clinging: Just as clouds form, shift, and evaporate, let thoughts arise and disappear on their own. See if you can notice gaps between thoughts.

6. Returning, always returning: The mind will try to hook you into tales and analyses. When you realize you've been swept away, gently and without judgment, escort your attention back to just watching the flow of thoughts like ever-changing clouds.

Recognizing Emotions Without Getting Caught Up

Emotions are more visceral than words; they carry an embodied charge. It's tempting to either avoid difficult emotions like fear, anger, or sadness or get submerged by them. Mindfulness offers a third option: acknowledging and holding our feelings with openness.

- Where in the Body?: When an emotion emerges, scan your body. Where do you feel it the most? Perhaps fear appears as tightness in your chest, anger as heat in your face, or sadness as a hollowness in your stomach. Simply recognize the sensations without trying to change them.

- Name to Tame: If helpful, find a single word that describes the core feeling: "fear," "anger," "sadness," "frustration." Labeling the feeling is like putting a signpost in the emotional storm, giving you a bit of perspective.

- Weathering the Wave: Recognize that feelings, like thoughts, are transient. They rise, peak, and fade. Ride the wave of the emotion, noting its changing intensity with curiosity instead of fighting it or spiraling into further reactivity.

- Compassion is Key: Be patient and kind towards yourself as you navigate emotional land. If you notice harsh self-judgment appear, try softening your inner voice: "This is hard," "This too will pass," "May I be gentle with myself."

Developing Non-Judgmental Awareness

The foundation of welcoming thoughts and feelings is a gentle attitude of non-judgment. Judging something instantly creates resistance towards it. We push away things we name "bad" and cling to those we deem "good". Mindfulness fosters acceptance of what is, allowing us to react more skillfully. Here's how you can develop this mindful quality:

- Notice the Judge: We all have an inner reviewer. The first step is becoming aware of that judging voice as it emerges. Does it analyze, compare, or catastrophize? Just watch this judgmental energy without identifying with it.

- "Good" or "Bad" are Just Labels: When a thought or emotion pops up, notice that any judgment (good/bad, pleasant/unpleasant) is something your mind adds on top of the raw experience. Focus on the bare emotions and feelings themselves.

- "Interesting..." as a Mantra: Replace harsh judgments with the phrase "Interesting...". Observe with fascination; notice how judgments create tension and tightness, while curiosity creates greater ease.

Here are two short guided meditations meant to support the practices covered in Week 3. I recommend recording them in your voice (using a phone app is fine) for a more unique experience.

Meditation 1: Thoughts as Clouds

Duration: 5 minutes

1. Find a comfortable sitting position where you can be alert yet relaxed. Close your eyes if it feels safe, or soften your gaze towards a neutral point.

2. Take a few deep breaths, noticing how the sensations of your breath anchor you in the present moment.

3. Now, as you continue breathing freely, open up your awareness to include the space of your mind. Picture a wide, open sky.

4. Notice thoughts arising, as if they are like clouds floating into view. Some may be small and fluffy, others big and dark. Some pass quickly, others stay.

5. Let your eyes rest lightly on this moving skyscape. No need to force anything, just watch.

6. If you find yourself completely carried away by a thought, that's perfectly normal. Simply smile inwardly and, without judgment, bring your attention back to the open sky of your mind.

7. Observe any subtle shifts that occur as you continue with this simple observation... perhaps a sense of spaciousness, lightness, or greater ease.

8. Before ending, acknowledge this moment of awareness you've made. Then gently re-connect with your real body and open your eyes when you're ready.

Meditation 2: Feeling the Wave of Emotion

Duration: 5 minutes

1. Settle into a comfortable position. Gently invite your eyes to close, or find a relaxed focus.

2. Begin by connecting with the feelings of your breath. This is your steady base throughout this practice.

3. Now, scan through your body slowly. Are there any areas where you feel tightness, tension, or any specific physical sensations?

4. Without trying to fix anything, see if you can locate any particular feeling – perhaps a subtle undercurrent of anxiety, a flash of frustration, or an echo of sadness.

5. Turn your mind towards the most present emotion. Where does it live in your body? Perhaps it has a shape, a warmth, or a heaviness. Simply observe.

6. Acknowledge the mood with a simple inner phrase, "Anger is here," or "I'm feeling some sadness."

7. If possible, stay with the sensations of the mood without getting lost in the story around it. Just like a wave in the ocean, notice how the feeling rises, builds, and then naturally dissolves.

8. If your thoughts wander, patiently return to the physical sensations. Use your breath as an anchor to stay centered in the present moment.

9. As you come to the end, know that emotions are fleeting visitors. Be kind towards yourself, and gently open your eyes.

Tips:

- Go Slowly: These are deceptively simple techniques. It's better to do a short practice well than to rush through it.

- Consistency is King: Short but regular practice builds 'mindfulness muscles much more effectively than rare long sessions.

- Don't Force Relaxation: Sometimes feelings will be intense. That's okay. Observe them as best you can. Acceptance rather than forced rest is the goal.

Remember: Practice, Not Perfection

Welcoming our thoughts and feelings can be the most difficult part of mindfulness practice, especially if there's a lot of internal turmoil. Be patient. Each try at non-judgmental observation plants a seed for greater freedom and peace in the long run.

WEEK 4: CULTIVATING KINDNESS

Having learned to anchor yourself in the breath, sense your body, and watch your thoughts and emotions, you're ready to infuse your practice with warmth and generosity of spirit. Developing compassion—both for yourself and others—is the heart of awareness. It changes our inner landscape, making us less brittle in the face of challenges and more receptive to joy.

Compassion and Self-Acceptance Meditations

Mindfulness isn't simply about being watchful or neutral. It's also about intentionally cultivating positive qualities like kindness, forgiveness, and understanding. When we are critical of ourselves and others, we feed stress, self-doubt, and disconnection. This week, we turn our attention inwards with kindness, paving the way for extending those same feelings outwards.

- Finding Space for Self-Compassion: Begin your meditation in your normal mindfulness posture, taking a few minutes to center yourself. Once settled, gently imagine a good friend who loves and accepts you completely. Visualize this friend radiating warm, comforting energy towards you. Notice what it feels like to be on the receiving end of this unconditional love.

- Softening the Inner Critic: Most of us deal with a sharp inner critic. With awareness, turn your attention towards any negative or self-blaming thoughts that might be present. Acknowledging their presence is the important first step. Slowly offer counterphrases to yourself: "This is difficult, but I am strong," "I am worthy despite my mistakes," "May I treat myself with gentleness." Let them echo without rushing.

- Embracing Difficult Emotions with Forgiveness: If, as you sit, difficult emotions rise – a pang of guilt, a flicker of shame – try holding them lightly and with self-compassion. Extend forgiveness to yourself for times of struggle or pain. You might think or say to yourself, " I forgive myself for past mistakes. I choose to act with kindness today." Focus on softening any tension or defensiveness you might feel, breathing into places of resistance.

Metta (Loving-Kindness) Phrases

The traditional practice of Metta includes directing well-wishes towards oneself, then progressively expanding the circle of compassion to others. It may feel a bit awkward at first, but stick with it, as the repetition plants seeds in your mind that grow stronger with time. Here's a simple script you can use, quietly or aloud:

Yourself:

- May I be safe?

- May I be healthy?

- May I be happy?

- May I live with ease?

A Loved One: Direct the same words towards a close friend or family member who evokes unconditional love in you.

A Neutral Person: Think of someone known but whom you don't know well – the barista at your coffee shop, someone you often see at the gym – and radiate those same positive wishes towards them.

A Difficult Person: This is where it gets truly changing. Can you offer those same good wishes to someone you struggle with? Don't force it, but allow a bit of softening. Perhaps wish not for immediate changes in your connection, but for their genuine well-being.

All Beings: Finish by visualizing all beings everywhere, human and non-human, and radiating boundless kindness. "May all beings be safe, may all beings be healthy, may all beings be happy, may all beings live with ease."

Dealing with Difficult Emotions with Gentleness

Even with a newfound openness and compassion, you will surely encounter challenging emotions while meditating (and indeed, throughout your day). Mindfulness in such situations involves:

- Acknowledging with Honesty: Rather than ignoring or suppressing unpleasant feelings, acknowledge them as a part of your present experience: "There is a lot of anger right now," or "This sadness is weighty." Allow these feelings to exist without attempting to modify or change them.

- Returning to the Body: Shift your attention to the physical feelings. Where do you feel the feeling primarily? Breathe into any places of stiffness or tightness. Observe their shape and texture, telling yourself that while uncomfortable, they are not dangerous.

- Softening: Can you add even a sliver of softness? This may look like relaxing your grip on a judgmental thought tied to the feeling or speaking to yourself with greater care. The softening may be subtle but consistent; with time, it can produce greater resilience.

Important Notes:

- Start gradually, extending compassion from sources of ease to areas of trouble without getting overwhelmed.

- Self-compassion takes work. Be patient with your inner judge

- The heart of these practices is in the real wishing for well-being, not simply mechanically repeating phrases. Tap into the feeling.

Here are a couple of choices for Week 4, focusing on compassion and metta.

Option 1: Short Self-Compassion Meditation (5 minutes)

- Settling in: Find your comfortable meditation position. Begin with a few deep breaths, letting your mind settle into your body.

- Invoking kindness: Gently bring to mind someone who loves and respects you – a friend, family member, spiritual figure, or even a beloved pet. Picture them looking at you with love and acceptance. Feel that sense of unconditional love flowing towards you.

- **Receiving kindness:** Allow yourself to be soaked in this feeling of warmth. Notice any feelings of softening or opening in your body. Let this sense of being cared for sink in.

- Offering self-compassion Now, slowly start repeating these sentences to yourself, allowing them to resonate deeply: May I be safe.

1. May I be healthy?

2. May I be happy?

3. May I live with ease?

- Difficult emotions: If difficult emotions or critical thoughts appear, recognize them. "There is sadness here," or "This is a moment of struggle." Extend love towards those parts of yourself: "May I be patient with myself," "I forgive myself." Breathe into areas of tightness or resistance.

- Return: As you near the end of the meditation, remind yourself that you can take this feeling of self-compassion into your day. Gently re-open your eyes.

Option 2: Guided Metta Meditation (10 minutes) (Follow the initial settling-in directions from the shorter meditation above)

- **Focusing on yourself:** Begin by offering these Metta phrases quietly towards yourself: May I be safe.

1. May I be healthy?

2. May I be happy?

3. May I live with ease?

4. Allow each phrase to settle in you, fostering a sense of well-being within.

- **Loved one:** Bring to mind someone you love and respect. Visualize them clearly and extend the same Metta phrases to them. Notice if any warmth or joyful feelings spread from your heart.

- **Neutral person:** Think of someone you see often but don't know well. Imagine sending them those same hopes for safety, health, happiness, and ease. Perhaps imagine the feelings radiating outward.

- **Difficult person:** (Proceed with care) If it feels right, bring to mind someone you struggle with. It may not be possible to wish them happiness right now. Perhaps start with "May they find peace," or "May their suffering lessen." Honor your limits.

- **All beings:** Gradually open the circle of your mind wider. Visualize your town, your country, the whole planet. Silently spread Metta to all beings everywhere: "May all beings be safe, may all beings be healthy, may all beings be happy, may all beings live with ease."

- **Return:** Gently shift your focus back to your body, your breath. As you finish the practice, carry a feeling of interconnectedness and generosity of spirit forward.

Tips

- Record your voice: Use your phone's voice recorder to make your own guided meditations to follow.

- Background music: Add soft, instrumental music if it helps create a soothing mood.

- Be flexible: You may find the time limits suggested don't work for you. Feel free to shorten or lengthen both of these practices to fit your needs.

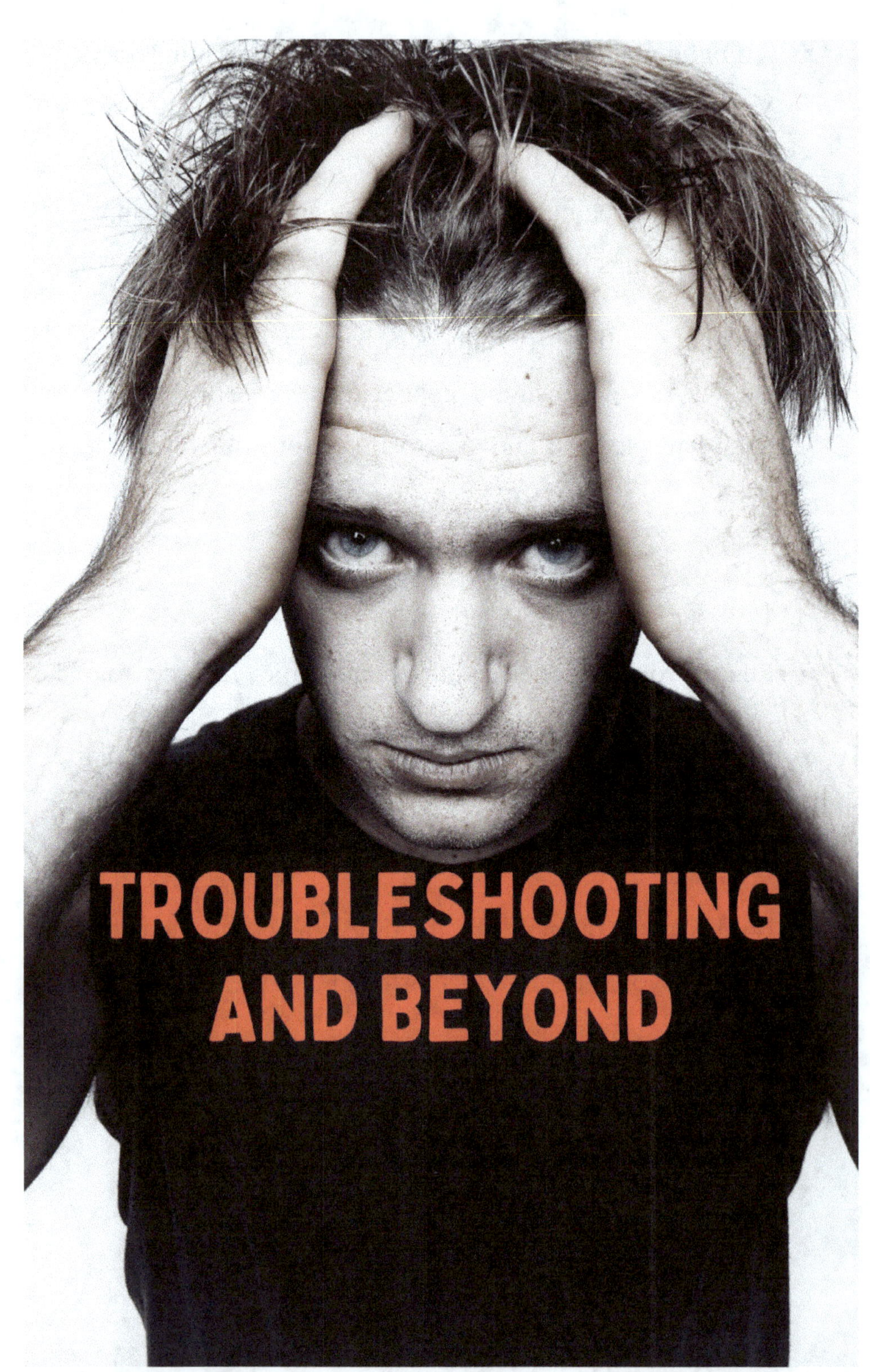

TROUBLESHOOTING
AND BEYOND

Chapter 4: Troubleshooting and Beyond

Common Challenges and How to Overcome Them

Even with the best of intentions and our handy 5-minute format, integrating mindfulness practice into your routine can bring up some obstacles. These bumps in the path are a sign that you're attempting, not failing. Let's look at the most common ones with instruments to manage them skillfully:

Challenge 1: Restlessness and Boredom

Why it Happens: Your mind and body, used to constant stimulation, might initially rebel against remaining still. Boredom may seep in, or an undercurrent of restlessness might make even a few minutes feel arduous.

How to Manage:

- Start Small: If remaining still for five minutes seems like torment, begin with just one or two minutes, progressively increasing the duration. Progress is preferable than giving up out of frustration.

- Get Physical First: Expelling some pent-up energy through exercise before your meditation may make that serenity later more accessible. Yoga or other meditative movement could also be excellent transitions into deeper contemplation.

- Shift the Focus: If the respiration feels too nuanced a focus, experiment with mindful walking, focusing on the sensations of your feet in contact with the ground. You can also concentrate on external sounds, a mindful cup of tea, or simply peering at a soothing piece of nature. This variety prevents monotony and provides an entrance point into cultivating presence.

- Acknowledge and Be Curious: If restlessness rises, merely acknowledge, "There is restlessness now". Observe it with fascination; how does it feel in your body? See if you can observe it with some detachment instead of allowing it to take over your experience.

Challenge 2: Intrusive Thoughts

Why it Happens: The mind is a thinking machine, so expecting complete silence within those initial few minutes is unrealistic.

Thoughts intrude; that's normal. The good news is that noticing those intrusions is mindfulness in action!

How to Manage:

- The Train Station Analogy: Think of your mind as an active train station with thoughts perpetually zooming in and out. Your task isn't to stop the trains but to station yourself on the platform and observe them arriving and leaving.

- Gentle Redirection: Each time you find yourself swept away by a thought, non-judgmentally label it "thinking" and then redirect your attention back to your breath. Do this over and over again with unwavering patience.

- Don't Take it Personally: We tend to identify significantly with our thoughts, regarding each one as an undeniable truth. Mindfulness encourages a sense of space: "Hmm, I'm having a thought that...", letting it float on by like a cloud rather than becoming fused with it.

- Use a Visual Anchor: Focusing on a flickering candle flame, a natural object, or your gentle rise and fall of the abdomen can all provide a stronger anchor from which to refocus when thoughts derail you.

Challenge 3: Judging Yourself for 'Doing it Wrong'

Why it Happens: When mindfulness is new, the inner critic loves to swoop in and declare: "This isn't working," "I suck at this," "I'm wasting my time." This self-judgment originates from not understanding how mindfulness actually functions.

How to Manage:

- Success Isn't Stillness: The goal isn't to attain some mystical state of zen-like serenity, particularly early on. True success resides in noticing when you've become distracted and tenderly returning to the present moment. Each "return" is a victory for mindfulness.

- Celebrate the Imperfections: Embrace those distracted moments as valuable data points; this is how your mind operates. Instead of condemning, be intrigued by what draws you away. Notice your customary thought patterns and the accompanying narratives. This information brings valuable self-awareness.

- The Practice Itself is the Goal: It's not about perfection but building capacity. Think of any talent – you get better at launching a tennis serve through repetition, even if initially, many balls fly erratically. Similarly, your ability to stay present strengthens with consistent practice.

- Self-Compassion as Your Shield: When judgments rear their head, simply label them, "There's judgment now". Treat these critical thoughts themselves as objects of investigation, then ameliorate them with kind reminders like, "I'm learning," or "This takes time and patience."

Important Reminders:

- Everyone Stumbles: Every single meditation teacher has labored with these very same challenges – this is part of being human!

- Progress, Not Perfection: Some days will feel smoother than others; that's normal. Instead of aiming for a flawless performance, emphasize regularity and a genuine commitment to the process itself.

- Seek Support: Guided meditations, applications, and community groups can be useful, reminding you that you're not alone.

Sitting for five minutes each morning offers profound benefits, but true mindfulness flourishes when translated into action. The more you imbue your daily activities with mindful attention, the stronger the neural pathways of awareness and self-regulation become. It's the difference between raising weights at the gym and integrating functional strength into your everyday posture and movements.

Mindful Moments in Everyday Life

Mindfulness needn't be confined to formal meditation time. Every activity offers an opportunity to practice being present and engaged. Here are some methods to introduce 'micro-mindfulness moments' throughout your day:

- Sensory Check-ins: As you proceed through your daily duties, consciously tune into your senses. While preparing your morning coffee, thoroughly heed the aroma, the warmth of the mug, and the taste on your tongue. This redirects your attention to the present, grounding you amidst autopilot tendencies.

- Transitions as Reminders: Transitions between activities are potent doorways to mindfulness. Instead of racing from a meeting to your workplace, use the walk as a mini-reset. Feel your feet connect with the ground, note your breath without altering it, and observe the changing environment around you. Turn routine transitions into pauses for presence.

- Chores with Presence: Often, mindless conversation dominates tasks like washing dishes or arranging laundry. Instead, consider intentionally transferring your attention to the tactile sensations involved. The temperature of the water, the texture of the fabric, the movement of your palms. Even apparently mundane duties become mini-retreats for the mind.

- One Mindful Activity Per Day: Pick one daily activity - consuming a meal, bathing, commuting - and commit to doing it with complete presence. Savor the tastes and textures of your food, experience sensations of water and soap during your shower, and observe your surroundings on your commute without letting your mind wander too far.

Walking Meditation

Walking meditation is a terrific bridge between seated practice and mindfulness in motion. It involves bringing focused awareness to the act of strolling. There are multiple variations:

- Barefoot Awareness: If feasible, locate a quiet patch of grass or smooth floor and walk barefoot. Pay close attention to the sensations of each step: contact between your feet and the ground, the elevating and swaying of legs, the subtle shifts in balance.

- Slow-Motion Walking: Slowing down the tempo helps focus your attention. This isn't a leisurely stroll: purposefully observe each aspect of a step – the heel lift, the weight transfer, the foot setting down. You can discover a comfortable rhythm but maintain that sensation of mindful movement.

- Outdoor Immersion: Walking outdoors adds another layer: sights, noises, and scents. Let your attention move like a gentle spotlight – the sensation of your steps, the breeze on your skin, the birdsong in the background – perpetually returning to the embodied experience of walking.

Integrating Mindfulness at Work

Modern workplaces are hotbeds of distraction and tension, making them an ideal arena to refine your mindfulness skills. These practices offer not only greater serenity but also enhanced focus and resilience:

- Pre-Meeting Mindful Minute: Before diving into correspondence or a congested meeting, take 60 seconds to center yourself. Close your eyes if possible, sense the support of your chair, and take a few mindful breaths. This straightforward act restores the nervous system and helps you step into the present with greater intention.

- Micro-Pauses during Work: Even if lengthier breaks aren't practicable, try integrating 30-second mindful pauses throughout your work. Pause typing, let your gaze soften, and take three deep breaths, noticing the rise and fall of your abdomen. These apparently trivial pauses accumulate, offering much-needed relaxation.

- strolling for Well-being: Instead of remaining desk-bound for lunch, consider a 10-minute mindful strolling break outdoors. Eat mindfully, if possible, and simply experience the fresh air and environs before returning to the workday.

- Mindful Emails: Before rushing through emails or launching emotional replies, consider pausing. Take a breath, feel your feet on the ground, and only then choose the appropriate tone and words for your response. This helps interrupt knee-jerk reactivity and cultivates a sense of presence even in communication.

Important Reminders:

- Start Small: Choose 1-2 methods to integrate mindfulness off the cushion, then progressively add more.

- Consistency is Key: Regular brief bursts are more effective than infrequent extended sessions.

- Be Kind When Distracted: The mind will wander! That's typical. Keep gently returning your focus to the selected task without self-judgment. Each return is a victory of attentiveness over default.

Here's a sample selection:

Mindful Eating Meditation (Approx. 3 minutes)

- Find a comfortable location with your selected food or supper set in front of you. Take a moment to connect with your respiration, allowing your body to calm.

- Begin by merely glancing at your food or snack. Notice the colors, the textures, and the distinct shapes. Appreciate the visual aspects as if you were seeing it for the very first time.

- Now, gingerly and with fascination, lift a portion of the food towards your nostrils. Allow yourself to completely imbibe its aroma. Are there any aromas that stand out? Any memories or associations that emerge?

- Slowly position a tiny bite in your mouth. Before chewing, just rest it on your tongue for a moment. Is there an immediate surge of flavor, a distinct texture?

- Start to swallow very methodically. With each swallow, observe how the texture changes, and how the flavor evolves. Can you identify various subtleties of taste?

- Swallow consciously, and note the sensation of the food traveling down your pharynx. Does it generate warmth or other sensations?

- Continue this mindful exploration of each morsel, letting go of haste or distractions. Simply be present with the experience of consuming.

Mindful Work Break (Approx. 1 minute)

- Step away from your computer or task at hand, if practicable. If not, just adjust your posture. Let your hands rest effortlessly in your lap or on your workstation.

- Close your eyes if comfortable, or let your gaze soften without focusing on anything in particular.

- Take a deep inhale through your nose, feeling your abdomen expand and ribs broaden. Hold your breath momentarily at the peak.

- Release the exhalation with a gentle exhale through your mouth, letting your shoulders relax down. Repeat this deep breath 2-3 more times.

- Simply observe the subtle sensations throughout your body – your feet anchored, your back against the chair, your palms at ease.

- Before resuming work, establish a concise intention. This could be something like "May I return to my tasks with clarity" or "May I work with presence."

Walking Meditation (Approx. 5 minutes)

- Find a space where you can walk comfortably for a few minutes. This can be indoors or outdoors. If feasible, remove your shoes for added grounding.

- Begin by standing erect, sensing the contact of your feet on the ground. Notice the distribution of your weight, and the subtle balance involved.

- With your first stride, focus on the lifting of your heel, the forward movement of your limb, the positioning of your foot back down. Maintain this slow and deliberate manner of strolling.

- Feel the subtle adjustments of balance, the contracting and releasing of muscles in your legs and pelvis.

- If your mind wanders, it will gently acknowledge the thought, and without judgment, return your focus to the physical sensations of each step.

- You can choose to focus solely on the act of walking or mindfully expand your awareness to include sights and sounds around you. Keep your attention mobile, observing without getting captivated by one single object.

- End by halting, again consciously sensing your feet connecting with the ground. Slowly open your eyes and resume everyday movement.

Important points:

- Use a Calm Voice: Your tone should be soothing and relaxed. Speak at a natural cadence, allowing for interruptions.

- Background Music (Optional): You can add light, instrumental music if it helps create a focused ambiance.

- Experiment: Try different variations, experiment with the durations of these meditations, and uncover what best supports your practice.

FINDING YOUR RHYTHM

While everyone can benefit from the fundamentals of mindfulness practice, there's no one-size-fits-all approach. To ensure this becomes a lifelong aid, it's vital to construct a routine that resonates with you. Here's how to personalize your journey:

- Timing Experimentation: Mornings offer consistency, but if they're genuinely impossible, locate another dedicated pocket of time. Perhaps during a break at work, an evening wind-down before bed, or even mindful micro-moments dispersed throughout the day. Listen to your own routines and prioritize what feels achievable.

- Duration Variation: While those focused 5-minute morning sessions provide potent results, don't hesitate to alter the length. You might add on to your morning meditations when time allows, or use short mindfulness check-ins amidst a chaotic day. Adjust length mindfully, considering your schedule and attention span.

- Explore Different Techniques: From breath focus and body scanning to walking and loving-kindness meditations, you've been exposed to numerous anchors and gateways to awareness. If one resonates profoundly, lean into it! Don't feel obliged to persist with practices that don't feel nutritious.

- Posture Matters: While traditional images elicit cross-legged immobility, mindfulness isn't dependent on one posture. Comfort is essential. You can sit erect on a chair, stand, or even lie down as long as alertness doesn't slide into sleepiness. Experiment and discover what supports your practice.

Resources and Support

Cultivating any new habit is supported by inspiration and community. The world of mindfulness offers an abundance of resources to nourish your journey:

- Apps: Apps are optimal for busy individuals. Options like Calm, Headspace, Insight Timer, and Ten Percent Happier offer brief guided meditations, timers, and even mindfulness courses. Explore their gratis offerings until you find one that suits your preference.

- Online Communities: Forums, subreddits, or social media communities dedicated to mindfulness provide connection and shared experiences. Exchange tips, discover accountability, and draw others' inspiration as you navigate this path.

- Local Classes or Workshops: If you seek deeper immersion or in-person learning, check out yoga studios, community centers, or Buddhist temples, often offering guided mindfulness classes and workshops. The energy of a group can be potent for cultivating the practice.

- Books and Online Articles: Deepen your understanding of mindfulness beyond these introductory chapters. There's a treasure trove of books investigating themes like self-compassion, navigating emotions, and specialized mindfulness for various applications (relationships, tension, etc.). Seek authors and instructors whose wisdom and style resonate with you.

Additional Tips for Personalization

- Keep a Mindfulness Journal: Jot down notes after your meditation sessions – how you felt, challenges that arose, or moments of insight. This record monitors your progress and exposes any patterns worth addressing for more enjoyable practice.

- Be Flexible: Some days will be simpler than others. Don't fall into the pitfall of all-or-nothing reasoning. A little mindfulness is better than none at all. Even if all you can muster is a single mindful breath, it counts!

- Share Your Journey: Inspire others and deepen your own comprehension by talking about your practice with friends or family. You might be astonished by their interest, generating positive ripple effects.

Important Note: While I can enumerate specific resources and offer suggestions, it's essential to do your own research. Explore different programs, teachers, and approaches until you discover something that genuinely clicks with you.

Mindfulness as a Personalized Adventure

Embracing mindfulness isn't about becoming a different individual or attaining a state of unachievable zen perfection. It's about establishing an empowering relationship with your mind, emotions, and your daily existence. As you personalize your practice, let inquiry, compassion, and the spirit of exploration be your guiding principles.

Your mindfulness journey began with a simple question: What if you could find greater calm and concentration within the whirlwind of your ordinary life? Throughout this book, you've discovered that such transformation is indeed possible, not in some distant retreat, but within the ordinary rituals that define your days.

These brief, targeted meditations have offered you much more than a few moments of stillness. With consistent practice, you've likely begun to notice:

- Reduced Stress: Your ability to ride the swells of challenges increases as you forge a non-reactive relationship with difficult thoughts and emotions.

- Enhanced Focus: Your attention has become a more disciplined instrument, less readily pulled off course by internal chatter or external distractions.

- Greater Self-Awareness: You've gained insights into your patterns, triggers, and interior reactions, opening the door to wiser choices.

- Increased Compassion: Cultivating compassion towards yourself helps mitigate judgment and fosters a more understanding connection with others.

- Moments of Joy: Simple activities, infused with presence, reveal layers of richness previously concealed by hurried and unthinking engagement.

This isn't about abrupt or profound transformation. Instead, those precious five minutes have been like droplets of water methodically shaping a stone. The cumulative effect of daily practice silently rewires your brain, altering your default way of processing the world. Remember, modest steps are consistently taken to lead to extraordinary destinations.

Mindfulness is an ongoing invitation, not a destination you reach and then mark off. There will be days when your meditation feels effortless, and days when the mind is particularly unruly. That's the nature of the practice. Be patient and trust that as long as you keep showing up, your awareness will progressively deepen.

Consider expanding your mindfulness toolkit as you move forward. Explore mindful movement practices like yoga or tai chi, investigate deeper forms of meditation, or look into mindfulness courses and workshops. There's always a place for further development and discovery.

The busiest individuals often realize they need mindfulness the most. Let those five minutes each morning be your non-negotiable anchor, a testament to your commitment to interior well-being. Think of that pause as an investment; throughout your day, you'll harvest the returns in heightened responsiveness, a tranquil heart, and a clearer perspective.

As you step back into the maelstrom of your existence, carry the essence of what you've cultivated on the cushion with you. Let every breath be a silent reminder of the tranquil power and spacious awareness available within you at any instant.